PALEO DIET

THE HOW–TO & NOT–TO GUIDE FOR BEGINNERS

ORLANDO SCOTT

Ash Publishing Inc.

ISBN 13: 978-1541198876

ISBN 10: 1541198875

Authored By: Orlando Scott

Edited By: William Smith

Cover design: Jamie Morton

BONUS: ULTIMATE DRINK RECIPE SERIES

Dear Reader,

Please visit www.ashpublishing.net/bonus1 to receive this gift I have prepared for you. In there, you will find over 186 drink recipes you can use to accompany any meal plan. There will also be very high quality and unique content included for the respective topics. I sincerely hope that this would be useful for you. Once again, thank you for purchasing this book.

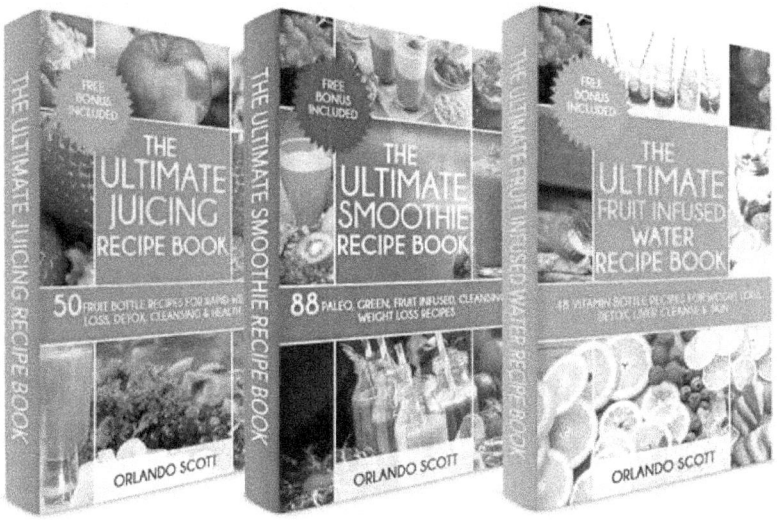

Table of Contents

Introduction

Are you on the lookout for a diet capable of delivering on its promise? Do you wish to develop a slim body just by making a few modifications to your existing diet? Well, you have come to the right place!

The Paleo diet is one of the best diets in the world and for good reason. Not only is it easy to follow, but stands head and shoulders above the others in terms of scientific backing.

It is an ideal diet to develop a lean and trim body; an aspect that ranks high on every person's radar. As you know, modern day lifestyles have pushed people's health to the limit, making it extremely tough to maintain a healthy body.

The need of the hour, therefore, is to stick with a healthy diet that aids in enhancing both physical and mental strength.

There are a plethora of diets available out there, all of which promise a different result. However, the Paleo diet actually delivers on its promise and lends you a healthy body. It is one of the most widely followed diets and ranks amongst the top 3 in the world.

This book will act as your guide to the Paleo diet and introduce you to a whole new world of fitness.

Let us begin!

Chapter 1:
History of the Paleo Diet

First and foremost, I wish to thank you for choosing this book and hope you have a good time reading it. In this first chapter, we will look at the history of the Paleo diet to understand the concept better.

The Paleo diet is now regarded as one of the best diets to follow owing to multiple health benefits that it imparts. Right from enhancing your physical stamina to increasing immunity, this diet promises a plethora of health benefits while almost always delivering them. But what started it all, and how did it manage to capture the attention of modern day health seekers? Well, let us find out!

The Paleo diet is one that mimics food choices that our ancestors made. The Paleolithic man walked earth billions of years ago and led a rather healthy lifestyle. In 1913, Joseph Knowles took on a hunter-gatherer style diet that mimicked what our ancestors ate. He is said to have been at the receiving end of a great deal of health benefits, thereby laying the foundations for the Paleo diet.

This prompted enthusiasm amongst dieticians and one doctor, in particular, Walter Voegtlin, began studying the diet in detail. Voegtlin is credited with coining the term "Paleo Diet," which first appeared in his 1975 book "The Stone Age Diet." The book managed to capture the attention of more and more doctors, and dieticians, who began their own experiments with the diet.

A decade later, Stanley-Boyd Eaton and Melvin Konner added to the works of Voegtlin thereby furthering the discussion on the diet and its effects on the body. However, it was not until 2002, when the diet accrued mainstream attention. One doctor Loren Cordain wrote extensively about it in his book, The Paleo Diet, which went on to become a big hit. The book described the Paleo diet in detail including its health benefits thereby prompting people to give it a shot.

Cordain, after developing interest, began to study the Paleolithic era, which lasted between 2.5 billion BC and 10,000 BC. He delved into details of the diet followed by people in the Paleo era and how it affected their bodies. In fact, he is now regarded as the father of the diet (not least for coining the term Paleo diet), for having introduced many of its concepts to the world. He understood that human genetic pattern has not changed over the course of time and remains intact. Over the course of 50 thousand plus years, the human genome has not changed any more than 0.2%, which is considerably low considering the effects of evolution on most other organisms. This phenomenon caused Cordain to come up with a diet that mimicked that of Paleo man.

It is no secret that modern day foods fail to have any positive effect on man's body and in fact, induce a negative effect. Not only do they introduce unnecessary chemicals, but also tamper with regular bodily functions. This, in the long run, is known to cause all types of issues in the body as well as expedite the onset of illnesses.

After understanding the diet's benefits and laying down the groundwork for the Paleo Diet, Cordain began prescribing it to his patients, in order to enhance their health. He was taken aback by the positive response and how the diet managed to improve the health of individuals that took it up. This prompted him to work further on the concept and make it palatable to modern day taste buds.

Paleo man depended on hunting and gathering techniques to avail day-to-day food. This meant that he only had access to meats such as fish and meats and fruits and vegetables. These formed his staple diet and did not have access to grains, seeds, lentils and the likes. These are therefore termed as modern day foods, incapable of being digested by modern man's delicate digestive systems.

The Paleo man led a healthy life free from illnesses. His organs worked optimally, and he possessed a very healthy bone structure. In fact, most of the remains that were found belonging to Paleo man were still intact, indicative of how his diet proved to be a true winner, in terms of up keeping a strong and healthy body.

Today, the Paleo diet is one of the most scientifically backed diets in the world. It is also one of the most searched terms on the Internet, thereby making it a very popular form of diet. In fact, it was the most searched word on Google in 2013, which catapulted its popularity making it a household name.

Its popularity was further enhanced when celebrities (Jessica Biel) and athletes (Kobe Bryant) began to endorse the effects of the diet and caused frenzy on social media. More and more people began taking it up and appreciated the effect that it has on the body.

The diet strongly urges people to return to the FOOD consumed by the Paleolithic man. Not only does it enhance overall health but also prepares the body to combat illnesses capable of damaging the body. This very fact has made it a winner amongst health enthusiasts and common people alike.

Its widespread acceptance is indicative of people wanting to change for the better, and leaving behind their bad food choices.

The diet is pretty simple to adopt and follow. You need not go through a complicated process to adopt it in your routine life. That being said, it is not your average "do as I say and you will be fine" diet and necessitates the adaption of certain lifestyle changes.

Through the course of this book, we will look at some of the basic concepts of the diet and delve into scientific details of its health benefits. There are expect clear instructions on the lifestyle changes to adopt and how best the diet can be made a part of your day-to-day life.

We will also look at a few recipes to try out and avail good health through the Paleo diet.

Chapter 2:
Modern Day Paleo Diet
vs. Original Paleo Diet

Modern day Paleo diet is quite similar to what our ancestors followed. Although it underwent a few changes, it more or less follows the same basic principles.

Here is looking at an overview of the foods consumed as per the diet. Before that, let us consider a few basic principles to bear in mind about the Paleo diet.

- The Paleo diet encourages the consumption of fresh foods that are free from additives and chemicals

- The basic structure of the diet is modeled around Paleo man's diet

- There is no proper guide detailing the portions allowed per meal. So it would be best to calculate it based on your body's daily calorie requirements

- The diet calls for the consumption of three healthy and nutritious meals per day

- The meals should be consist of the basic food categories as described under

The Paleo diet focuses on three main components of food namely proteins, multivitamins, and fats.

Lean proteins

Lean proteins make up for a large part of the Paleo diet. Proteins assist in the build up of muscles, maintain bone health and enhance immunity. Paleo man had access to meats that were free from chemicals. He would hunt down small animals such as rabbits and deer and consume the meat raw. He also scavenged for leftovers left behind by other animals.

It is, of course, not possible for you to go hunting for your meat, especially in this day and age where everything is commercialized. The best option is to settle for free range meats, which come closest to what Paleo man accessed. Free-range meats come from farms where animals are allowed to roam and graze freely. They are not fed chemical laden fodder that ultimately ends up affecting human health. They are made to graze on green lands containing fresh grass. The meat from these farms is much better quality wise and richer in essential nutrients.

These meats can be found in the organic section of the supermarket. If you fail to find them there, then look for a butcher who sells free range meats. If you are up for it, then consider raising your livestock to avoid looking for it outside.

Organic free-range eggs are also a must to incorporate into your Paleo diet. Eggs are full of proteins and will introduce a world of goodness to your body. Raising your chicken will help you remain with good quality free-range eggs.

Meat should make for a large part of every meal you consume. Poultry such as chicken and duck are good options as they impart lean proteins. Red meats such as goat and venison are rich in iron and will assist in enhancing your blood quality. Seafood is highly recommended, as the meat is soft and nutritious. Assign each meat to a different day so that you manage to sample every type within a week.

Proteins serve the purpose of filling you up in a way that prevents you from feeling hungry between meals. You need not worry about hunger pangs that can leave you feeling groggy. The meals will give your body substance and make you feel fuller after eating a regular meal.

Paleo man had strong and lean muscles courtesy of lean proteins. These muscles aid in keeping fat at bay and also impart strength to the body. As old age approaches, these muscles stabilize the body and provide support. The body tends to slow down after reaching 50 and so, will be best to develop and maintain muscle mass right from an early age. Adopting the Paleo diet can ensure the same and prepare the body for old age.

The Paleo diet does not cater to non-vegetarians alone. Although it can appear so owing to the encouragement of meat consumption, there are a lot of options for vegetarians in the protein department. Some of the protein-rich foods include nuts such as almonds and pistachios, spinach leaves, and broccoli.

Fruits and vegetables

Fruits and vegetables are just as big a part of the Paleo diet as meats. Paleo man is said to have hunt down many animals to extinction thereby necessitating the need to turn to other sources. Fruits and vegetables made for an easy choice, as they were available in abundance.

Paleo man picked fresh fruits such as berries, apples and bananas directly from the trees and consumed them fresh. Modern day Paleo dieters who prefer to pluck fruits straight from trees follow this ideology. That way, you access nutrients faster and avail their direct effect on the body.

If you are unable to do so, then shop for organic produce. Organic fruits are grown in a natural environment without the use of chemicals. If you are unable to find any in your area, then look for them online.

Growing your produce is also an option if you cannot find fresh organic fruits. A small patch of land will be enough to grow seasonal fruits.

Vegetables, like fruits, form a big part of the Paleo diet and are meant to provide the body with essential nutrients. As with fruits, Paleo man had direct access to quality vegetables. He pulled out tubers from the ground, plucked out fresh beans, carrots, beetroots, etc.

Organic works here too, as it is important to consume foods that are free from chemicals. Once again, shop for them at an organic market or consider growing some of your own.

A large part of your diet should consist of fruits and vegetables. Around 40% of your meal should be made up of it as it imparts great health. A good idea is to make the plate as colorful as possible. This means you pick out vegetables and fruits that are of different colors and add them to your plate. That way, you have access to many different nutrients capable of enhancing good health.

Paleo man did not have access to fire and therefore did not cook anything. Now extending this philosophy can prove to be quite hard, as our bodies are accustomed to consuming cooked foods. Continue to cook foods like you usually, do. However, it will be a good idea to cook it at low temperatures, as it maintains nutritional levels.

A crockpot is a handy product to buy as it cooks food at ideal temperatures. Add the ingredients to it and leave them for 6 to 8 hours.

Fats and oils

The third main component of the Paleo diet is fats and oils. These are used to cook with as they are laden with nutrients. Rich in omega 3 fatty acids, they are meant to help enhance heart and brain health. They also contain vitamins such as A and E that are important for the upkeep of the body.

Nut and seed oils also contain saturated fats, but a lot of misconception prevails over the health benefits provided by these fats. However, both monounsaturated and polyunsaturated fats aid in lowering cholesterol levels in your heart. This means it will be easy to control the bad cholesterol in your systems just by consuming healthy fats and oils.

Some of the best oils to pick include olive oil, sunflower oil, and coconut oil. MCT oil is also a great option, as it is light and healthy.

Fats and oils are used to cook the vegetables and meats. They are also used as dressing for salads. Flavored oils such as chili infused oil can be used to add to soups.

These form the three main food groups that form a part of the Paleo diet. Apart from these, spices and herbs are also a part of the diet. They are used to enhance the flavor of food and make it more palatable.

The list of acceptable food as per the diet is mentioned as under

Meats

- Poultry
- Turkey
- Chicken breast
- Pork tenderloin
- Pork chops
- Steak
- Veal
- Bacon
- Pork
- Ground beef
- Grass-fed beef
- Chicken thigh
- Chicken leg
- Chicken wings
- Lamb rack
- Shrimp
- Lobster
- Clams

- Salmon
- Venison steaks
- Buffalo
- New York steak
- Bison
- Bison steaks
- Bison jerky
- Bison rib eye
- Bison sirloin
- Lamb chops
- Rabbit
- Goat
- Beef jerky
- Eggs (duck, chicken, goose)
- Pheasant
- Quail
- Lean veal
- Chuck steak

Fish and seafood

- Bass
- Salmon
- Halibut
- Mackerel
- Sardines

- Tuna
- Red snapper
- Shark
- Sunfish
- Swordfish
- Tilapia
- Trout
- Walleye
- Crab
- Crawfish
- Crayfish
- Shrimp
- Clams
- Lobster
- Scallops
- Oysters

Vegetables

- Asparagus
- Avocado
- Artichoke hearts
- Brussels sprouts
- Carrots
- Spinach
- Celery

- Broccoli
- Zucchini
- Cabbage
- Peppers
- Cauliflower
- Parsley
- Eggplant
- Green onions
- Butternut squash
- Acorn squash
- Yam
- Sweet potato
- Beets

Nuts and Oils

- Coconut oil
- Olive oil
- Macadamia oil
- Avocado oil
- Grass-fed butter

Nuts/ Seeds

- Almonds
- Cashews
- Hazelnuts
- Pecans

- Pine nuts
- Pumpkin seeds
- Sunflower seeds
- Macadamia nuts
- Walnuts

Fruit

- Apple
- Avocado
- Blackberries
- Papaya
- Peaches
- Plums
- Mango
- Lychee
- Blueberries
- Grapes
- Lemon
- Strawberries
- Watermelon
- Pineapple guava
- Lime
- Raspberries
- Cantaloupe
- Tangerine

- Figs
- Oranges
- Bananas

Chapter 3:
Foods to Avoid During the Paleo Diet

The Paleo diet bans the consumption of certain foods that were not available to Paleo man. They were not exposed to these foods and relied solely on whatever was available to them. Here is looking at some of the foods that are banned from the diet and why you must avoid consuming them.

Dairy products

Dairy products are not allowed on the diet. Paleo man was not exposed to them, as he did not rear cows and other milk-producing animals. He was not aware of its existence and thus did not consume any dairy. It was not a part of his dietary intake, and so, you must avoid consuming it as well.

As per studies, milk is capable of inducing asthma in certain people and so, will be best to stay away from it. It is also known to induce allergy related illnesses such as celiac, which affects your digestive system and leads to loose motions. Just by giving up on dairy products, you can both enhance your overall health and improve well-being.

Dairy products include milk and all its derivatives including butter, ghee and the like. However, there is an option to replace these with products made from nut and seed milk. This includes almonds, cashew nuts, etc.

Make your own by looking up the recipes online. They will contain the same goodness as milk and prevent your body from being denied basic nutrients.

Here is a list of banned dairy as per the Paleo diet.

- Butter
- Cheese
- Cottage cheese
- Non-fat dairy creamer
- Skim milk
- 2% milk
- Whole milk
- Dairy spreads
- Cream cheese
- Powdered milk
- Yogurt
- Pudding
- Frozen yogurt
- Ice milk
- Low-fat milk
- Ice cream

Legumes and grains

Legumes and grains were not available to Paleo man. They were exposed to fruits, vegetables and meats alone, and did not consume lentils, grains, etc. This only means that you too will have to stay away from them, as your systems will not be in a position to digest these easily. Studies have shown that long-term use of these can lead to stomach issues that will compromise good health.

If you are accustomed to consuming these, then it will take some time for your systems to make the change. You need to remain patient with your body and give it time to make the adjustments. It will, especially, be difficult for those who exposed to such foods right from a young age, but a little effort will go a long way in avoiding their consumption.

Here is looking at the different legumes and grains to avoid on the Paleo diet.

- Cereals
- Bread
- English muffins
- Toast
- Sandwiches
- Triscuits
- Wheat Thins
- Black beans
- Broad beans
- Fava beans
- Garbanzo beans
- Horse beans
- Kidney beans
- Lima beans
- Mung beans
- Adzuki beans
- Navy beans
- Pinto beans

- Red beans
- Green beans
- String beans
- White beans
- Peas
- Black-eyed peas
- Chickpeas
- Snow peas
- Sugar snap peas
- Miso
- Lentils
- Lupins
- Mesquite
- Soybeans
- Tofu
- All other beans
- Crackers
- Oatmeal
- Cream of wheat
- Corn
- Corn syrup
- High-fructose corn syrup
- Wheat
- Pancakes
- Hash browns

- Pasta
- Fettuccine cheese
- Lasagna

Soft drinks and juices

Soft drinks and juices are also prohibited as per the Paleo diet. It is obvious that Paleo man did not have any access to these and thus, you too should remain as away from it as possible.

But it is understood that you will have a tough time as most of us are far too used to consuming these on a regular basis. The only way to stop consumption is by making an effort and replacing it with healthier options. These options include fruit infused water, lemonades, fresh fruit juices, etc. With time, it will get easier as your body will crave these more than aerated and other soft drinks.

Apart from soft drinks, all sugar-laden juices are also prohibited and will require you to stay away from it.

Here is a list of banned drinks

- Coke
- Sprite
- Pepsi
- Mountain Dew
- Apple juice
- Orange juice
- Grape juice
- Strawberry juice

- Guava juice
- Mango juice
- All other store bought ready juices

Sugar and artificial sweeteners

Paleo man did not have access to sucrose. He only consumed fructose that was available through fruits. Sucrose is directly linked to the onset of diabetes and other endocrine illnesses. It is, therefore, important to stave off consuming it as much as possible.

Taking small steps towards it will help with the process. This includes avoiding sugar during morning tea/coffee, reducing consumption of sweets, etc. Even if it is a gradual process, you will have to put in the necessary efforts. There can be times when you have no choice. During such times, garner control over the portion of serving and limit it to as less as possible.

Apart from sugars, Paleo man did not have access to any artificial sweeteners. They will end up adding to your calories and increase fat. Here are some of the ones to avoid.

- Acesulfame potassium
- Sweet One
- Sunett
- Aspartame
- APM
- Equal Classic
- NatraTaste Blue

- NutraSweet
- Aspartame-Acesulfame salt
- Cyclamate
- Not in the US as per FDA
- Calcium cyclamate
- Sucaryl
- Erythritol
- Sugar alcohol
- Zerose
- ZSweet
- Glycerol
- Glycerin
- Glycyrrhizin
- Licorice
- Hydrogenated starch hydrolysate
- Sugar alcohol
- Isomalt
- Sugar alcohol
- ClearCut Isomalt
- Decomalt
- Hydrogenated Isomaltulose
- Isomaltitol
- Lactitol
- Sugar alcohol
- Maltitol

- Sugar alcohol
- Maltitol syrup
- Maltitol powder
- Hydrogenated High Maltose Content Glucose Syrup
- Hydrogenated Maltose
- Lesys
- Sweet Pearl
- Mannitol
- Sugar alcohol
- Neotame
- Polydextrose
- Sugar alcohol
- Saccharin
- Acid saccharin
- Equal Saccharin
- Necta Sweet
- Sodium Saccharin
- Sweet N Low
- Sweet Twin
- Sorbitol
- Sugar alcohol
- D-glucitol
- Steviol glycoside
- Rebiana
- Sucralose

- NatraTaste Gold
- Splenda
- Tagatose
- Natrulose
- Xylitol

Junk food

Paleo man was not even remotely exposed to any form of junk foods. It is modern man's bane and a must for you to keep away. Junk foods are laden with fats and chemicals that can negatively impact your health and jeopardize normal functioning. They will also tamper with your mental makeup and prevent your body from functioning optimally. It will pay to limit consuming junk foods and gradually stop it completely.

Here is a list of junk foods to avoid

- Burgers
- Hot dogs
- Junk pizzas
- Fries
- Other junk foods

Processed foods

Processed foods are also banned from the Paleo diet. They are laden with sugars and other chemicals not easily digested by the body. MSG or Monosodium Glutamate is one of the most dreaded of them as it is capable of altering your bodily functions. It also kills your appetite for healthy foods thereby further damaging your health.

Studies have a shown link between junk food and the death of healthy brain cells. This is another major cause for concern, especially for those who consume these foods on a regular basis.

If it is tough to stop consuming these, then try coming up with alternate options that can be prepared within the confines of your kitchen. Replace all the unhealthy ingredients with healthier options within the limit of the diet.

Here is a list of junk foods to avoid consuming when on the Paleo diet

- Pretzels
- Chips
- Triscuits
- Wheat Thins
- Cookies
- Sun Chips
- Pastries

Apart from these, you have to stay away from any other processed foods that can contain sugars and chemicals.

Smoking/alcohol/drugs

It is very obvious that Paleo man did not have access to cigarettes, drugs or alcohol. He led a chaste life free from any such mood altering substances. Although drugs tend to make you happy momentarily, by increasing the dopamine content, they end up releasing a lot of cortisol in the brain. This leads to stress, which leads to binging.

Cigarettes can lead to the onset of lung diseases. If you are an addict, then join a rehab to deal with the issue. It will be best to keep these at bay and focus on the diet at hand.

Here is a list of alcohol to avoid

- Beer
- Wine
- Vodka
- Gin
- Rum

Chapter 4:
Health Benefits of the Paleo Diet

The Paleo diet is one of the most scientifically backed diets in the world and imparts a whole world of goodness. Here is looking at its top health benefits and what makes it one of the best diets in the world.

Cell health

Cells are possibly the most important parts of the human body. They keep the organs in shape and provide the body with necessary energy. One of the key components of cells is saturated and unsaturated fat. These fats need to be balanced out, to maintain cell health. Polyunsaturated fats are found in abundance in red blood cell membranes.

The Paleo diet is one that introduces to the body both saturated and unsaturated fat, in the right ratios. The diet encourages the consumption of foods rich in omega 3 fatty acids, which enhance cell health. Eicosapentaenoic acid (EPA) and docosahexaenoic acid (DHA) form two of the main components of omega 3 acids. They enhance the function of brain cells and protect them from oxidative damage. The diet also aids in enhancing the regenerative function of cells. Regeneration assists with the formation of new and healthy cells capable of functioning optimally.

Brain health

The Paleo diet helps maintain brain health. It contains nutrients capable of increasing cognition and maintaining basic cell health. The diet has proven its use in the case of Alzheimer's disease. It is a degenerative illness that mainly occurs during old age. The omega 3 fatty acids in the diet form a barrier against the degeneration of cells thereby preventing the onset of the illness. It is also known to reduce its effects on health. Apart from Alzheimer's, it also helps with other mental illnesses such as dementia. This too mostly occurs during old age and causes a rapid decline in cognition. Cognition refers to the uptake of information and its synthesis. Consuming fresh water fish such as trout and salmon ensures proper brain development. Vegetarians can pick flax seeds as it provides a healthy dose of omega 3 fatty acids.

Lean muscles

Lean muscles help in replacing the fat in your body. Lean muscles refer to new muscles that replace the older ones. These are harder to burn and will lend the body support. They form after regular muscles tear and give way to leaner ones. Once these new muscles form, they end up shrinking down the fat cells. Once they shrink, they will not allow fat to be deposited in the body. The Paleo diet encourages the consumption of protein-rich foods. These proteins aid in the development of lean muscles and encourage the depletion of fat cells.

Healthier guts

Guts are very essential for the upkeep of a healthy body. Not only do they assist the liver in purifying the blood but also regulate the release of hormones. Consumption of modern day foods laden with sugars and other chemicals only leads to a condition known as the leaky gut syndrome. This can cause the gut to leak out thereby causing discomfort. One of the best ways to deal with the situation is getting on the Paleo diet. The foods consumed through the diet will ensure good gut health. They also reduce inflammation in the gut, which is caused due to modern day foods. The nuts and seeds in the diet will help enhance overall gut health.

Multivitamins

It is a well-known fact that the body thrives on multivitamins. These vitamins help in keeping the body strong and enhance overall well-being. The Paleo diet encourages the consumption of fruits and vegetables of different colors. Each one consists of a different set of vitamins and minerals that contribute towards enhancing the different parts of the body. As a rule of thumb, try to cook 2 cups of vegetables per meal per person. This will help the body avail the daily requirement of nutrition. A good sample of vegetables includes carrots, beetroots, spinach, kale, peas and cauliflower. Mushrooms too help in adding to the body multiple vitamins as also proteins.

Digestion

The Paleo diet helps with better digestion. As you know, mimicking our ancestors' food choices helps with better break down of foods. This maintains digestive health and keeps the systems healthy. The diet encourages the consumption of many types of gut healthy foods that contribute towards maintaining the digestive tract clean and healthy. Metabolism also considerably improves. This means that the person will be able to digest and eliminate faster before giving the body a chance to store fat.

Allergies

As per studies, people who take up the Paleo diet suffer from lesser allergies. This means that they manage to keep away from certain allergy-inducing foods such as milk and grains. Milk is said to lead to asthma in certain people, and avoiding it can help in staving off its onset. This will successfully enhance good health and improve overall well-being.

Weight loss

The Paleo diet helps with weight loss. Weight loss is an issue that bothers many people. But only a few manage to control it and develop a lean body. One good way of doing so is by taking up the Paleo diet. It controls the intake of unwanted foods capable of affecting the body in a negative manner. Once you take up the diet, you will see that the fat is dissolving and leaving your body. The diet is known to cause this and help with maintaining a slim and athletic body.

Immunity

The Paleo diet helps in strengthening immunity. Immunity helps fight away illnesses and improves blood circulation in the body. The foods consumed as per the diet all work towards enhancing overall well-being. People who consume the Paleo diet succeed in staving off the onset of minor illnesses such as common colds and fall sick less often. The liver is strengthened by the diet thereby boosting immunity and increasing resistance to illnesses.

Skin/hair health

Skin and hair health is of utmost importance to most people, especially women. As we age, skin tends to lose elasticity and develop wrinkles. This can adversely affect the image and also make the person conscious. But with the Paleo diet, it is easy to maintain your youthful glow. The diet prescribes the consumption of healthy foods containing vital nutrients such as vitamin e and folate. Both of these contribute towards keeping the hormones in check, which is a major contributor towards remaining youthful. The proteins in the diet help add elasticity to the skin and also strengthen hair follicles. You will notice your hair has turned healthier and shinier. It will also improve the tensile strength thereby reducing breakage.

Diseases

Adopting the Paleo diet can ensure reducing the onset of modern day illnesses. This includes the likes of certain types of cancers that can be brought about by the consumption of junk and processed foods. It is very important to stick closely to the diet's prescription to stave off the onset of illnesses. As per studies, people who avoided consuming these modern foods were able to keep all such illnesses at bay and develop a strong body free from complications. You too can have the same by sticking with the Paleo diet.

Diabetes

One of the biggest precursors to the onset of diabetes is consuming junk foods. Those who keep away have the chance to reduce its onset to a large extent. Diabetes mostly occurs through insulin resistance. Insulin controls the breakdown of sugar in the body. When you hit the body with sugary and fatty substances, it ends up confusing your body and making it difficult to break up the sugars. The Paleo diet helps in taking away from the burden and reduces the work performed by your liver. With time your body will be in a position to remain resistant.

Chapter 5:
Why Adopt the Paleo Diet?

The Paleo diet is designed to help people enhance their living and make the most of their life. Just like Paleo man, people can enhance day-to-day living and improve their overall well-being.

Here are some of the reasons to adopt the Paleo diet and reel in a healthier life.

Fit life

Life is precious and is no secret that all of us try to live it to the fullest. But many factors come in after a certain point that make it difficult for us to lead a fit life. Some of these include stress and consumption of junk foods. These can lead to the onset of mental and physical issues. The best way to combat these is by taking up an effective diet. There are many diets out there all of which promise different results. However, there is one that offers and delivers on its promise. The Paleo diet is one of the best in the world and will help you see results in no time at all.

Fitness is a challenge these days. People hardly find time to focus on their health and indulge in activities that are good for the body. The Paleo diet, however, ensures you consume foods that enhance your health and make way for a fitter lifestyle.

Longevity

The Paleo diet has been proven to increase longevity. The diet, much like the Mediterranean diet, focuses on the consumption of healthy foods and leaves out foods that can damage the systems. This, therefore, leads to a longer life free from illnesses. But as is with other diets, it is important to keep up with it and not give up on it as soon as you start seeing results. The diet should be viewed as a lifestyle choice and not just a fad diet. With time, you will see that the diet has become an active part of your life and can make lifestyle modifications as per its requirements.

Ease

The Paleo diet is fairly easy to adopt and will leave you with lasting results. One does not have to make too many modifications to the existing diet, especially those who are already following the vegetarian or began the diet. The diet can be transitioned into within a few days and maintained for life. In fact, its ease is what makes the Paleo diet one of the most preferred around the world. A good start would be to maintain a record of your progress so that you know exactly how you are faring.

Happier life

It is obvious that leading a healthy life is going to make you happy. The diet has been designed to enhance your overall life and make it well worth the effort. Your stress levels will come down and help you reel in a calm mindset. This will go a long way in enhancing your overall well-being.

Productivity

Enhancing productivity leads to a better life. Your energy levels will increase and help you make faster decisions. It will reflect in your workspace and leave you feeling good about yourself. Carrying a healthy homemade meal that in keeps with the diet will help you look forward to it during office hours.

Passing on genes

If you accustom your body to the diet, then you will be able to pass on some of the good genes to the future generations. This will especially be feasible if you start with the diet at an early age and continue with it for life.

Chapter 6:
FAQs About the Paleo Diet

When you start a new diet, it is obvious that many questions will cross your mind. In this chapter, we will look at some of these questions and attempt to answer them successfully.

Why should I pick the Paleo diet?

The Paleo diet is now well-renowned thanks to the results that it provides. The diet has been proven on the grounds of science, and will almost always deliver on its promise. The diet is easy to follow and will leave you feeling healthy from the get go. The Paleo diet is suitable for a large audience and will make a great choice, even if you are trying a diet for the first time. In fact, once you start with it, you will not turn to any other diet. The diet is easy to stick with and can turn into a lifestyle choice.

How does the Paleo diet work?

The Paleo diet taps into a person's genetic makeup and aims at strengthening the person's core systems. Modern day foods have contributed towards a decline in the health of the general public, and the best way to solve the issue is by turning to a diet followed by our ancestors. They did not have any access to the foods that we are now exposed to and therefore lead a healthier life. The Paleo diet works on this very simple principle and enhances the body's disease-fighting capacity, thereby rendering longevity. It leaves out all the ingredients that can punish good health including fats, sugars, and trans fats.

How is it different from other diets?

The Paleo diet is unique and unlike others out there. It is the only one that mimics the food choices that our ancestors made and leaves a person feeling strong and healthy. The diet is backed by many scientific theories (some of which are cited through the course of this book) and will surely help a person see feasible results. It lays emphasis on the consumption of fresh fruits, vegetables and meats alone, which is unique.

Is it suitable for a vegetarian to take up?

Yes. The diet is suitable for a vegetarian to take up. There are not too many impositions regarding the fruits, vegetables, and herbs that can be consumed as per the diet. Vegetarians and vegans can both take up the diet as it leaves out the consumption of dairy products, as they were not available to Paleo man. The diet is designed to suit the palate of a wide range of people and will make a great choice for vegetarians to take up.

Why does it leave out fiber rich foods?

The Paleo diet follows the food choices that our ancestors made and promotes the consumption of only those foods that were easily available to him. This means that it will leave out grains, legumes, and other such fiber-rich foods. However, the diet promotes the consumption of foods that are rich in fiber such as meats and leafy vegetables.

Can I take it up to build a lean body?

Yes. The diet will make a great choice for all those looking to develop a lean and muscular body. It is designed to promote the consumption of foods that are rich in proteins. These will help you build up a muscular body with the presence of lean muscles. However, it will have to be supplemented with regular exercise to avail maximum benefits.

Is the food going to be bland?

Not necessarily. The diet promotes the consumption of herbs, spices and other such natural condiments that render a dish flavorsome. They can be added in any desirable quantity to heighten the taste of the dish. It is understood that most of us are used to consuming junk and processed foods that are loaded with chemical flavors. But with time, your palate will adjust to the taste of the diet and will stop feeling bland.

Are there any precautions to observe?

As is with any other diet, you might have to observe a few precautions before taking up the Paleo diet. These will be mentioned in a later chapter of this book. They are simple precautionary measures that can be followed with ease.

Didn't Paleo man live a short life?

This is one of the most frequently asked questions about the Paleo diet. Many people wonder as to how the diet can be a healthy one when Paleo man himself lived a short life.

However, this is only a misconception, as Paleo man did not live a short life. He had an average lifespan but was free from illnesses. He mostly succumbed to being eaten by bigger animals, as he could not defend himself against them. So the Paleo diet is a good one to follow to develop a healthy body free from illnesses.

How long will results take to show?

That will depend on your body type and how much effort you are putting into the process. Some people tend to see fast results owing to putting in a good level of effort into it, whereas some others will see slow results owing to putting in lesser efforts. Following a plan and recording your progress from time to time will help you not just stick with the diet but also see faster results.

These form some of the common questions that get asked on the Paleo diet. I hope you found a feasible answer to your questions.

Chapter 7:
Sticking with the Paleo Diet

Many people tend to take up a diet and abandon it halfway through. This will not only confuse the body but also nullify any of the positive effects accrued through the diet. It is, therefore, important to stick with the diet to avail its full benefits.

Here are a few tips to follow to keep up with the Paleo diet.

Schedule

The very first thing to do is make a timetable. Working with one helps in keeping track of the meals you consumed, the exercise routine you took up, etc. A simple timetable mentioning the different activities against appropriate times will ensure that you eat your meals on time as also get some physical activity. There are many apps available now that help you prepare a timetable. You need not keep changing the whole thing and just modify the meals and exercise routines. Having a hard copy of it serves as a reminder to stick to the schedule.

Shopping

The next step is to go shopping. Try to shop every morning for fresh produce. Going and getting it yourself will motivate you to eat healthy. Make a list of the produce to buy so that it becomes easier for you to shop. If it is too much of a hassle to shop them at the store, then order them online. Many websites sell organic produce and will deliver them to you within scheduled time. This also helps you stave the temptation of visiting processed food aisles and picking up something forbidden by the diet.

Overhaul

Overhaul the kitchen and fridge. Do away with all the foods banned by the Paleo diet and make way for the foods to eat. Make a list and go shopping for it. The best idea is to have a friend help out. That way, you will get done faster and be able to dispose of some of the unwanted foods. If there remain excess, then it can be donated to soup kitchens. Try to get rid of as much of the old food as possible including processed and junk foods. This will go a long way in helping you stick with the Paleo diet for longer.

Appliances

Certain appliances can make your work easier. Cooking a Paleo meal can get a little monotonous at times. The best way to deal with this problem is by making use of a crock-pot. Also known as a slow cooker, it helps in cooking the meal at a slow pace. This ensures uniform cooking and retains the nutritional value of the food. Just add the ingredients to the pot and allow it to cook on low for 8 to 12 hours. This is perfect to cook breakfasts as you can add the ingredients at night and have your breakfast ready in the morning. Another appliance to buy is the pressure cooker. This serves the opposite purpose of a slow cooker. It cooks the food at a faster pace by using steam. A spiralizer will help you make noodles out of vegetables. These will replace your regular wheat and non-wheat noodles.

Recipe books

Making use of recipe books can also help you stick with the diet better. This book will provide you with a few recipes that can last you a month. Similarly, a good cookbook containing Paleo recipes will help you keep going. You won't have to go looking for new dishes and can try out a new recipe every day. Once you get the hang of it, you will be able to create recipes of your own. Get your family members involved with the cooking process and make anyone person's favorite meal per day.

Role model

It pays to have a role model and emulate him or her. It can be anybody including a favorite athlete or an actor. If that is too far-fetched, then look within your family. There will be a lot of inspiration there, capable of making you stick with the diet. Having a poster of them will inspire you to put your best efforts and try to come close to their figure. If you are taking up the diet for other causes then having a visual reminder of them can help with sticking to the diet.

Partner

Taking up the diet with a partner can go a long way in helping you stick with it. The partner can be a friend a sibling or your spouse. The two of you can keep reminding each other about the diet and eating the right meals. It also helps during the exercise routine, as it will serve as an inspiration to have a partner workout with you. Couples yoga is a good choice, as it will make the workout interesting. The two can also take turns in the kitchen to cook up a Paleo meal.

Group

If you do not find a partner, then there is the option to join a group. A Paleo dieters group will consist of other people working with the diet. Not only can you find a partner there but also avail expert advice from people who have tried and tested the diet. If you were unable to find any such group in your area, then it would be a good idea to start one by yourself. Advertise it on your social media platform to garner an audience. Hold regular meetings to discuss topics about the diet. Encourage people to exchange useful tips that can help you and the others.

Record

Record and measure your progress. Every time you find an inch of waist less or a couple of pounds lesser, it will motivate you to continue with the diet for a longer time. Buy yourself a scale to keep a tab on your weight and a tape to measure your statistics. These will give you a glimpse of how much weight you have lost. But do not obsess over it and give your body some time to lose weight at its own pace. Set a few deadlines and try to reach the goal within that time.

Reward

A reward can help motivate you to keep up with the good work. A reward can be anything like a material reward or a relaxing massage. As long as you feel rewarded for the good work, it will enhance the output. But make sure you do not reward yourself with a cheat meal. It will work counterproductively to the diet. Also, bear in mind the frequency of the reward. If you reward yourself too often, then it will lose its value. Stick to rewarding yourself every 2 months or so, or after you hit a milestone.

Carry meals

One of the biggest problems faced by dieters is visiting a restaurant with friends and family. It becomes a little difficult to look for a place that serves Paleo food. In such a case, the best thing would be to carry your meals. Carrying your meals will ensure you do not have to sit at the table empty handed. Enjoy your Paleo meal while the rest enjoy their food.

Heads up

It will be a great idea to tell everybody in your life about the diet so that they prepare themselves to host you. This is especially important for parties so that they can, prepare Paleo meals for you. Give them a list of foods that you eat so that they can prepare the meals accordingly. If it is too much of a hassle, then you can always carry your meals. Invite friends over and throw them a Paleo party. That way, you have the chance to give them a glimpse of what you consume on a regular basis.

Profess

A fail proof method to stick with the Paleo diet is to profess about its benefits. Start a blog and capture your journey. If you have taken it up to lose weight, then update your progress from time to time. Create a social media profile to do the same. That way, you will have the chance to garner support for your endeavor. However, prepare yourself for any of the negative comments that might come your way. You cannot exercise control over them and must learn to ignore them.

These form some of the lifestyle modifications to make when you take up the Paleo diet. As mentioned earlier, it might seem like a daunting task to overhaul your diet. However, do not be intimidated by it and take it up with passion.

Chapter 8:
What Not to do During the Diet

The Paleo diet is comparatively an easier one to adopt. However, there are some basic rules to follow when you take it up, to avail its full benefits. Here is looking at some of the things to avoid doing during the Paleo diet.

Overeat

One of the first and foremost things about the diet is not to overeat. Many people assume that since the diet only promotes the consumption of healthy foods, it will be a good idea to increase the portion per meal. But this is not true and will work counter-productively. Ensure that you control the portion per meal. Come up with a plan that will help you consume the right amount per meal. Some good tricks to achieve this is to make use of smaller plates and bowls to eat your meals. Use a measuring cup to measure out the ingredients that will be used for cooking the meal. Leave out the last two bites per meal and wait to check if you feel satisfied with the meal. If you do, then reserve it for the next meal.

Add-ons

Be careful with the add-ons. The diet forbids the consumption of condiments such as sauces, as they are laden with chemicals. So don't tempt yourself into adding them to your foods assuming they will be nullified by the goodness of the diet. You have to prepare yourself to consume foods that are only encouraged as per the Paleo diet and stay away from any such add-ons. If you are used to them and cannot break the habit, then it would be best to prepare some by yourself. Use recipes that make use of natural ingredients and lie within the boundaries set by the Paleo diet. Put them in the same bottle so that you automatically reach for them during meals.

Skip meals

Do not make the mistake of skipping meals, as it will affect your diet, and body, in a negative manner. You must aim at having all your meals on time to ensure that the body has time to break it down efficiently. If you have skipped a meal, then don't try to make up for it by overeating the next one. Instead, try to consume a snack that will supplement the meal. The breakfast is the most important meal of the day and should never be skipped. Consume one that is high in protein and rich in fiber. A standard breakfast can contain eggs and a small piece of whole-wheat toast that helps in maintaining the balance of nutrients.

Liquid calories

Be careful with the amount of liquid calories that you consume. Not many realize that liquids too can add calories to the body. These can come from smoothies, juices, and other such beverages. Although the Paleo diet does not restrict the consumption of these, it will be important to measure the intake of calories. If in case you are unable to modify the calorie intake with the liquids then balance it out by modifying the calories in the meals. By adding low-calorie ingredients such as kale and lettuce to smoothies, you successfully bulk it up and reduce the amount of calories per serving.

Cut out fat

Do not make the mistake of cutting out fat from the diet. The diet bans the consumption of dairy but not that of fat. Our bodies require a little fat from time to time to remain lubricated from the inside. So make use of butters extracted from nut and seed milk. These will help with keeping the body healthy from the inside. It is a myth that the consumed fat is converted into fat inside the body and gets stored there for a long time. As long as you time your meals and consume a fatty meal just before your workout, your body will have a good chance of burning it away. Make a list of fats and their calorific content and consume it accordingly.

Over salty

Salt is a great seasoning to add to meals as it uplifts the flavor. However, over salting your meals can cause the meal to lose some of its goodness. Salt can lead to hypertension and increase your blood pressure. A better way of seasoning food would be to make use of herbs and spices. These will lend the dish a unique flavor and make it tasty. Keep a bottle of oregano on the table so that you reach for it, during a meal, as opposed to a bottle of salt. If the meal has ended up being too salty, then use a potato to reduce the salty flavor in the dish.

Stress

One of the biggest mistakes to avoid making during the diet is undertaking stress. Stress has the tendency to overwork the body. The mind ends up releasing cortisol, a chemical that can slow down the body considerably. It is, therefore, imperative to keep stress at bay and avoid undertaking activities that can lead to it. Another good way to avoid stress is by taking up a therapeutic activity. This can be meditation or something that diverts your mind. Exercising helps with controlling stress to a large extent. It promotes the release of serotonin in the mind, a hormone responsible for inducing happiness. This will help you remain happy and give the diet a chance to work well on your body.

Lose sleep

Sleep is of utmost importance for the body. When we sleep, our body goes to work and repairs everything from the inside out. It works on repairing the tissues, muscles and everything else that needs to be restored. By not sleeping enough, we deny our body the chance to heal itself. Try to clock a minimum of 8 to 10 hours of sleep, as it will restore your systems. Cut down on watching television or using the laptop before sleeping as it can affect your sleep cycle. Instead, listen to some soothing music that will work on your mind and relax it. Stay away from stressful activities before hitting the bed to enhance your sleep.

Over exercise

Do not over exercise as it can lead to stress. Even if you are in a hurry to lose weight, it will be best to stick with whatever your body is comfortable with and used to. Exercising in the mornings is better than in the evenings as you will be quite energetic and be in a position to burn away more fat. However, if you are unable to exercise in the mornings then can also take it up in the evenings. Stop as soon as you cannot exercise more. Pushing your body beyond that point will only lead to aches and pulls.

Lose interest

Many people tend to take up the diet with a lot of enthusiasm and then rapidly lose interest. This can be a bad thing, as the full benefits of the diet cannot be availed. It will, therefore, be best to remain enthusiastic until you reach your end goal. Abandoning the diet half way through will not only nullify your hard work but also make it tough for your body to adapt to the sudden change. If, for some reason, you are unable to continue with the diet then discontinue it slowly. Jumping into your old food habits will only affect you negatively. Once you are ready to take it up again, start on a slow note.

These form the different things to avoid doing during the Paleo diet. It is very important to do so to enhance the effects of the diet on your body.

Chapter 9:
Basic Exercise Routines to Adopt

It is not enough for you to rely on diet alone to lose weight. It has to be supplemented with exercise to avail its full benefits. Paleo man led a very active life. There was no television and other such distractions and spent most of his time hunting and walking. This made way for a toned body with lean muscles and very little fat. But the same cannot be said about modern day man. We hardly get any physical activity that leads to fat. It is, therefore, important to get as much exercise in as possible to beat the fat.

Here is an exercise routine that can help you attain your desired weight loss goals.

Cardio exercises

Cardio exercises refer to those who get your heart rate up and burn away the fat in your body. This is a great type of exercise for those who want to target the stubborn fat. Cardio exercises can be of many different types. Based on your body type, pick the one that works best for you. Here is looking at some of the different types.

Cycling

Cycling is a great way to avail full body exercise. It can elevate your heartbeat within a short period. Cycle in the mornings and try to go as far as possible. Having a partner always helps as the two of you can keep each other company and ride as far as possible.

Running

Running is the easiest and most effective form of cardio. It gets your heart rate up in no time at all and starts working on your fat deposits. Again, run in the mornings so that you have the chance to put all your energy to good use. Running for 30 minutes is going to help your cause in a big way. If you don't have time in the morning, then run in the evenings. Again, find a partner to remain motivated.

Swimming

Swimming is preferred over some of the other cardio exercises since it is easier to take up and faster to lose your weight. You will not feel too stressed or worked up. 20 laps will go a long way in shaping your body.

Stepping

Stepping involves using a stepper. This helps in toning your obliques and also strengthens your core. If there is no stepper, then use a staircase and move up and down.

Dance

Dancing is a great little way to lose weight and maintain a toned body. Pick a dance routine that is capable of working on all the different areas of your body. Belly dancing is regarded as one of the best ways to loosen the stubborn stomach fat.

Rowing

Rowing is a good way to burn away fat. A rowing machine will help you work on your arms, thighs, calves and obliques. All it takes is a rowing machine and some high-energy workout.

Crunches

Crunches are performed after cardio exercises since they help with toning the stomach muscles and make them firmer. There are many types of crunches to choose from including basic crunches and bicycle crunches. You must feel a burn when you take these crunches up and be in a position to tone your body.

Remember to always do some warm up before taking up cardio exercises. Warming up helps in preparing the body for the workout. A few squats will do the trick.

Weight training

Weight training is undertaken to build muscles and work on arm fat. Pick weights based on your capacity. Lift them after cardio exercises, as that is the best time to push your body into losing weight and developing lean muscles. Basic lifts need to be mixed with advanced ones so that your muscles are thoroughly flexed.

Yoga poses

Yoga poses are some of the best forms of exercise for your body. They are not too demanding and will work on your entire body. They mostly work by massaging your internal organs and shaping them up. Here is looking at some simple poses to adopt.

Triangle pose

The triangle pose is pretty simple and helps tone your abs. Stand straight and look forward. Now split your legs a little and place your hands on your hips. Tilt to one side and place your palm against the opposite foot. Rise again and repeat it on the other side. Keep this going until you feel a good burn.

Downward dog

The downward facing dog is a great pose to take up when you wish to flex your back muscles. Start by sleeping face down on the floor and look ahead. Now place your palms in front of your head and lift yourself up. Support your lower torso with the help of your toes and your upper torso with your fingers. Remain in the position for as long as feels comfortable. Slowly lower yourself down and then repeat the position.

Lotus pose

The lotus pose is a relatively simple pose but is quite effective in toning your stomach and thigh muscles. Sit on the floor and fold your legs such that they cross each other at the ankles. Placing opposite feet on your thighs will be ideal. Straighten your back and place your palms on your knees. Maintain the pose as long as possible to train your muscles and tone them up.

Cobra pose

The cobra pose works on toning your stomach muscles. It is a relaxing pose that frees tension in your lower back. Sleep on the floor with palms next to your face. Now keep your legs glued to the floor and lift your upper body up. Look upwards and maintain the pose for a few minutes before releasing.

Yoga is both simple and effective and the perfect choice for those who do not want to overwork themselves.

CrossFit training

CrossFit training is a heavy-duty exercise routine that requires you to put in a lot of effort. Better known as interval training, it involves indulging in some heavy duty exercising before taking a break and then continuing once again. Keep doing so until your body feels a burn and then rest.

There are many workout routines to choose from ranging from full body to body specific ones.

Each routine is referred to as workout of the day and helps you target one specific part of your body.

Pick out simple workouts that can help your entire body. For example, the ANNIE workout requires you to perform 21 thrusters followed by 21 pull-ups followed by 15 thrusters followed by 15 pull ups followed by 9 thrusters and finished by 9 pulls ups. You must try to finish this as soon as possible without taking too many breaks in between. It will initially feel a little tiring but get better with time.

Pick a new routine every time so that it does not get monotonous. Introduce variety into the whole regime so that it helps tone your body thoroughly.

Pilates

Pilates are the next best exercises to perform. They include taking up slow exercises that work on the entire body. They work on the internal muscles and tone them up. It is pretty simple to take up Pilates and will suit a wide range of people. It is one of the best ones to pick for women looking to tone their bellies and burning away fat.

Carve out a regime based on your body type and whatever suits you best.

Chapter 10:
Meal Plans for the Paleo Diet

Here is a simple 1-week meal plan for you to follow.

Monday

Breakfast- Start your day with a filling mushroom sandwich (recipe provided). Mushrooms are rich in proteins and also vitamin D. this balances out the lack of dairy as per the diet. They are also loaded with selenium, which keeps your digestive and urinary tract clean.

Lunch- lettuce wraps (recipe provided) are both light and tasty. It makes use of simple ingredients and is loaded with nutrition. The wraps are easy to make and light to carry. They will not be too imposing to prepare for a weekday.

Dinner- End your Monday with a simple yet fresh chicken salad (recipe provided) that can be whipped up in a matter of minutes. Keep all the ingredients ready in the fridge and assemble them to make the fresh salad.

Dessert- lemon pie bars (recipe provided) are easy to make and delicious. Lemon is full of anti-oxidants and will make your body stronger. Make a large batch and store in the fridge for a week or so.

Snack- zucchini chips are yummy snacking options. They are rich in multiple nutrients and will make for extremely tasty snacks. You will not have to worry about the calories, as they are light on the stomach.

Tuesday

Breakfast- Start the day with Paleo breakfast rolls (recipe provided). It takes very little time to bake these and can sit in the oven while you get ready for work. The dry fruits in the role will keep you energetic and healthy all through the day.

Lunch- Paleo noodles (recipe provided) are easy to make and quite delicious. The noodles, in this case, refer to zucchini noodles that are spiralized. The Paleo diet bans consumption of any other forms of pasta and so; this makes for a great recipe to include in your diet.

Dinner - A fresh salad made from cashews and broccoli (recipe provided) will help keep you fit. It makes use of simple and fresh ingredients that are easily available in your fridge. It can also be saved for breakfast the next morning.

Dessert- Paleo coconut bars (recipe provided) are tasty and unique. They are easy to make and taste great. Make a medium sized batch and keep in the fridge for 2 to 3 days.

Snack- Spicy chia seeds (recipe provided) are easy to whip up. Those who love jalapenos will love this recipe as it mixes pumpkin with jalapeno peppers and leaves you with a tasty snack.

Wednesday

Breakfast- Sweet potato filled with eggs (recipe provided). Sweet potatoes are rich in vitamin A and C and will nourish your body thoroughly. It also contains many minerals such as manganese and copper, which improves body composition.

Lunch- a Mexican lunch (recipe provided) will keep it interesting. It makes use of fresh ingredients that are full of vital nutrients. It is easy to put together and will leave you with a tasty meal.

Dinner- a shrimp salad (recipe provided) will make for a great dinner option, especially after a heavy Mexican lunch. The salad is fresh and will leave you feeling full. You can customize it to your liking and enjoy a tasty meal.

Dessert- Paleo doughnuts (recipe provided) are a great choice for the midweek. It is easy to put together and will make for a great dessert.

Snack- eggplant chips (recipe provided) are a good one to settle for. It is easy to make and tasty.

Thursday

Breakfast- Start off your day with a Paleo French toast (recipe provided). French toast makes for a wholesome meal that will fill you up. It combines with the goodness of bananas that are loaded with iron. This will make for a healthy and nutritious meal.

Lunch- The BLT sandwich (recipe provided) is a big hit as it makes use of fresh seasonal ingredients. The Paleo version is healthy and tasty. It calls for just a few ingredients and can be easily assembled on a busy workday.

Dinner- Whip up a simple dinner burger (recipe provided) to satisfy your palate on a Thursday night. The burger uses simple ingredients but will leave your taste buds wanting more.

Desserts- Key Lime pie (recipe provided) is a favorite among all and one that is sure to be a hit with anyone. This simple Paleo key lime pie is simply superb and will make for a fantastic dessert option.

Snack- Apple nachos (recipe provided) are a tasty snack to make. Apples are filled with nutrients and will keep you alert and active all through the day.

Friday

Breakfast- Paleo breakfast pudding (recipe provided). Who doesn't love a sweet dish for breakfast? The Paleo breakfast pudding is just the one for all those who wish to satisfy their sweet tooth. It is made from fresh ingredients that will keep you feeling full and energetic until lunchtime.

Lunch- Fish is one of the most preferred Paleo ingredients owing to its health benefits. It provides the body with omega 3 fatty acids that help maintain heart health. A simple fish salad will make for a light and tasty meal.

Dinner- the Paleo pizza (recipe provided) makes for a great choice for a Friday night. It is extremely easy to make and should not take you any more than an hour. It makes use of fresh easy to find ingredients that will make a delicious pizza.

Desserts- who doesn't love cake? The Paleo cake (recipe provided) is simple and easy to put together. It will make a great cake for everyone, including those whose aren't following the diet.

Snack- Paleo crackers (recipe provided) are easy to bake. It only takes a few ingredients and can be stored for a week or two.

Saturday

Breakfast - 1 pot potato, bacon (recipe provided). This dish is simple to make and will require just one pot. The bacon will lend your body proteins, and the potatoes will increase vital nutrients. The eggs make this dish a healthy one to add to your daily diet.

Lunch- Lamb patties with mint chutney (recipe provided) makes for the perfect lunch on a Saturday afternoon. It will prove to be a treat as it is quite tasty. Lamb will provide your body with iron and mint will cool your systems down. It makes for a winning combination and will tingle your taste buds.

Dinner- End the day with a creamy chicken curry (recipe provided). Although it will take time to prepare, it will make for the perfect recipe for a Saturday night meal.

Dessert-Paleo cranberry cookies are easy and great. They can be put together using just a few ingredients. In fact, they leave our flour and make for an easy and innovative recipe.

Snack- sweet potato chips (recipe provided) are easy to make and taste great. They can be made in advance and stored for a month.

Sunday

Breakfast- Paleo pancakes (recipe provided). Pancakes make the best choice for lazy Sunday mornings. These pancakes combine the freshest ingredients and leave you with mouthwatering pancakes served with a delicious berry sauce.

Lunch- The Thai salad (recipe provided) is easy to assemble and tasty. The ingredients are simple to put together and will make for a good brunch option. Make them in mason jars and throw your friends a Paleo party.

Dinner- If you wish to continue the party into the night, then whip up some Paleo pork chops (recipe provided). These pork chops are sweet, sticky and delicious. They are easy to make and can be prepared in no time.

Dessert- baked banana (recipe provided) is very simple to make and make for a tasty treat for a Sunday.

Snack- Filled avocados (recipe provided) is a good choice for a snack. Easy to put together and full of flavor.

Chapter 11:
Simple Paleo Breakfast Recipes

Mushroom Sandwich

Ingredients

- 1/2 lb Bacon

- Avocado, chopped

- Lettuce leaves

- 2 Portobello Mushrooms

- 1 teaspoon oil

- Pepper to season

- 1 teaspoon all-spice powder

- Almond meal burger

Instructions

1. Heat a pan and toss in the sliced bacon strips.

2. Remove the bacon and allow its juices and oils to remain in the pan.

3. Slice the bread into halves and place it on the pan.

4. Allow it to soak in all the oils and juices and roast well.

5. Add the oil to the pan and toss the halved Portobello mushrooms.

6. Allow it to soften.

7. Season with pepper.

8. Assemble the sandwich by placing the burger bun on a plate.

9. Arrange the lettuce leaves on top.

10. Add the mushrooms over it.

11. Place the bacon strips and cover with the bun.

12. Sprinkle the all-spice powder over it to enhance the flavor.

13. Serve hot.

Paleo Breakfast Rolls

Ingredients

Dough

- 2 tablespoons coconut oil
- 1 small egg
- 1 tablespoon honey
- 1 teaspoon vanilla extract
- 1 1/2 cups almond flour
- 1 teaspoon baking soda
- 1 teaspoon salt

Filling

- 1 tablespoon cinnamon powder
- Honey, for drizzling
- 1/4 cup dates, chopped
- 1/4 cup walnuts, chopped

Drizzle

- 2 tablespoons honey
- 2 tablespoon coconut cream
- 1 teaspoon cinnamon

Instructions

1. Preheat the oven to 325 degrees Fahrenheit.

2. Add the oil to a bowl along with the eggs, honey and vanilla and mix until well combined.

3. Run the flour, baking soda and cinnamon through a sieve to well combine.

4. Now mix the flour with the wet ingredients and whisk until well combined.

5. Mix it into a soft dough and roll it onto a wax paper.

6. Use a rolling pin to flatten out the dough.

7. Add the cinnamon, walnuts, honey and dates to a bowl and mix until well combined.

8. Smear it over the roll and spread using a spatula.

9. Now gently roll the dough tightly by wrapping the wax paper.

10. Once it becomes a tight roll, cut it into bite sized rolls.

11. Place on a greased baking tray and place in oven for 10 to 15 minutes.

12. Once done, serve hot.

Potato Filling

Ingredients

- 2 sweet potatoes
- 1/2 breakfast sausage
- 4 eggs
- 1/4 cup half and half
- 2 tablespoons mayo
- 2 teaspoons mustard
- 1/3 cup half and half
- 1/4 cup shredded cheddar cheese
- Fresh cilantro leaves to sprinkle

Instructions

1. Preheat the oven to 350 degrees Fahrenheit and place the sweet potatoes on a baking tray.

2. Bake for an hour or until the potatoes completely soften.

3. Add the sausages to a pan and allow it to cook.

4. Add the eggs to a bowl along with the half and half and whisk until well combined.

5. Add in the mayo, mustard and cheese and mix well.

6. Scoop out the centers of the sweet potato and add it to the egg mixture.

7. Add the mix to a pan and allow it to scramble.

8. Place the scramble in the center of the potatoes and serve hot with a sprinkling of fresh cilantro leaves on top.

Paleo French Toast

Ingredients

- 3 medium bananas
- 1 1/2 cups roasted cashews
- 1 cup almond flour
- 2 tablespoons coconut oil
- 2 eggs, beaten
- 1 tablespoon honey
- 1 teaspoon baking soda
- 1 teaspoon baking powder
- 1 teaspoon vanilla extract
- ½ teaspoon cinnamon
- Pinch of salt

Toast

- 2 eggs
- ⅓ cup coconut milk
- 1 teaspoon vanilla extract
- ¼ teaspoon cinnamon powder
- 2 tablespoons coconut oil

Instructions

1. Preheat the oven to 375 degrees Fahrenheit.

2. Add the cashews and coconut oil to a blender to make a smooth paste.

3. Add in the bananas to the mix and make a smooth paste from it.

4. Sieve the dry ingredients together to well combine.

5. Mix in the dry ingredients with the wet and make a smooth batter.

6. Add to a greased tray and place in the hot oven for 25 to 30 minutes or until the bread rises.

7. Once done, allow it to cool down.

8. Add the bananas to a bowl along with the honey and mix until well combined.

9. Add it on top of the sliced bread and serve hot.

Paleo Breakfast Pudding

Ingredients

- 6 dates, quartered
- 1 can coconut milk
- 1 tablespoon vanilla extract
- 2 -cups fresh raspberries
- 8 Tablespoons chia seeds

Instructions

1. Add the dates, coconut milk, vanilla extract, and raspberries to a blender and mix until well combined.

2. Add the chia seeds to a blender and make a fine powder.

3. Add the smoothie to a glass and sprinkle the seeds on top.

4. Serve chilled.

5. You can add in some fresh fruits on top to make it a fruity smoothie.

One Pot Potato Bacon

Ingredients

- Cilantro leaves to 12 ounces bacon, cut into strips
- 1 tablespoon coconut oil
- 5 cups sweet potatoes, chopped
- 4 cups zucchini, chopped
- 1 cup onion, chopped
- 1 red bell pepper, chopped
- 5 large eggs
- Black pepper to taste
- sprinkle

Instructions

1. Preheat the oven to 400 degrees Fahrenheit.
2. Add the bacon to a skillet and allow it to crisp up.
3. Remove the bacon and allow the fat to remain back.
4. Add the additional oil to the pan and toss in the potatoes.
5. Once they soften. Add the onion, zucchini and bell pepper and mix until well combined.
6. Cover and let it all cook.

7. Toss in the bacon and mix.

8. Add the eggs on top and allow them to cook as it is.

9. Once the whites harden sprinkle the pepper on top.

10. Serve with a sprinkling of cilantro leaves on top.

Paleo Pancakes

Ingredients

- 5 large eggs
- ½ cup coconut flour
- ½ cup almond flour
- 1 cup full-fat canned coconut milk
- 1 tablespoon honey
- 1 teaspoon white wine vinegar
- 1 teaspoon vanilla extract
- ½ teaspoon baking soda
- Pinch of salt
- 1 teaspoon coconut oil

Berry sauce

- 1 cup raspberries
- 1 cup blueberries
- 1 cup blackberries
- 1 tablespoon honey
- 1 teaspoon arrowroot flour

Instructions

1. Add the eggs to a bowl along with the coconut milk, vinegar, vanilla and coconut oil and mix until well combined.

2. Add the flours and baking soda to a sieve to well combine.

3. Add the wet ingredients into the dry ingredients and whisk until well combined.

4. Heat a griddle and add in the coconut oil.

5. Place a ladleful of the batter on it and allow it to brown on one side before flipping and browning on the other.

6. For the sauce, heat a pan and add in the raspberries, blueberries, blackberries and honey and mix until well combined.

7. Once it starts becoming runny, add in the arrowroot powder to thicken it.

8. Serve by drizzling the sauce on top of the pancakes.

Chapter 12:
Simple Paleo Lunch Recipes

Lettuce Wraps

Ingredients

- 1 pound beef, ground

- 2 tablespoons coconut oil

- 1 medium onion, chopped

- 1 large green bell pepper, chopped

- ½ teaspoon salt

- 1 teaspoon black pepper, freshly ground

- 1 teaspoon cumin powder

- ½ teaspoon cinnamon powder

- 1 cup tomatoes, chopped

- ¼ cup sultanas

- 2 tablespoons green olives, chopped

- 2 tablespoons capers

- 2 tablespoons olives

- ⅓ cup red onion, chopped

- ⅔ cup tomatoes, chopped

- 2 tablespoons cilantro, chopped

- 2 teaspoons fresh lemon juice

- Salt to taste

- Lettuce leaves

- Cooked brown rice

- Parsley to sprinkle

Instructions

1. Heat a griddle and add in the beef to it.

2. Stir occasionally and allow it to soften.

3. Add oil to a pan and let it heat.

4. Stir in the onions and cook until soft.

5. Add the tomatoes and mix until well combined.

6. Toss in the garlic, salt and pepper and mix.

7. Add the olives and capers and mix until well combined.

8. Allow everything to come together into a thick mix.

9. Cover and cook for 10 to 12 minutes.

10. Serve hot with a sprinkling of fresh parsley leaves on top and some brown rice on the side.

Paleo Noodles

Ingredients

- 3 cloves garlic, chopped

- 3 tablespoons butter

- 20 jumbo shrimps, deveined

- 1 teaspoon paprika powder

- 1 teaspoon cayenne powder

- 1/2 tsp Himalayan sea salt

- 1 teaspoon red pepper flakes

- 1 teaspoon garlic, chopped

- 1 red onion, chopped

- 2 large zucchinis, spiralized

- 1 red pepper, chopped

- 1 tablespoon butter

- Fresh parsley to sprinkle

Instructions

1. Spiralize the zucchini to make thin noodles.

2. Add the shrimp to a bowl along with the seasoning and mix until well combined.

3. Add the butter to a pan along with the garlic and brown it.

4. Toss in the onion and pepper and mix until well combined.

5. Add the shrimp and allow it to crisp up.

6. Toss in the spiralized zucchini to the mix and stir until well combined.

7. Add in the salt and pepper and mix until everything comes together.

8. Add some butter on top to help the noodles slide.

9. Serve with a sprinkling of fresh parsley leaves on top.

Paleo Mexican Lunch

Ingredients

- 3 small carrots
- 1 big sweet potato
- 1 tablespoon taco seasoning
- Salt to taste
- 1 teaspoon olive oil
- 1 chicken breast
- 1 tablespoon honey
- Salt to taste
- 3 roma tomatoes, chopped
- 1 red onion, chopped
- 1 lemon, juiced
- 1 jalapeño pepper, chopped
- Pepper to taste
- 1/2 avocado, chopped
- Baby spinach, chopped
- 4 fried eggs
- Parsley to sprinkle

Instructions

1. Peel the carrots, potatoes and cut them into bite-sized pieces.

2. Toss in the seasoning and mix until well combined.

3. Preheat the oven to 250 degrees Fahrenheit.

4. Add the fries to a baking tray and bake in the oven until crisp.

5. Add oil to a pan along with the chicken and cook until brown.

6. Add in the seasoning and honey and mix until well combined.

7. Add the tomatoes, jalapeno and onion and mix well.

8. Add in salt and combine.

9. Fry the eggs in a pan to your liking.

10. Serve the dish hot with the egg on top and a sprinkling of fresh parsley on top.

Paleo BLT Salad

Ingredients

- Lettuce
- 1 large avocado
- 2 handfuls of cherry tomatoes
- Half a cucumber
- ½ cup cilantro leaves
- 4 rashers of bacon
- 1 cup feta cheese
- 1 tablespoon olive oil
- 1 tablespoon mustard
- 1 lemon, juiced
- 1 tablespoon balsamic vinegar

Instructions

1. Add the bacon to a pan and allow it to crisp up.
2. Meanwhile, cut everything into small pieces and add to a bowl.
3. Sprinkle the feta on top and mix until well combined.
4. Add it to a serving bowl and add the bacon on top.

5. Mix the oil, mustard, lemon and vinegar in a bowl and drizzle on top of the salad.

6. Serve cold.

Fish Salad

Ingredients

- 4 ounces baked salmon
- 4 cups assorted greens
- 1/2 cup zucchini, chopped
- 1/2 cup raspberries
- 1 tablespoon balsamic glaze
- 2 tablespoon olive oil
- 1 teaspoon sea salt
- Pepper to taste
- 1 tablespoon thyme leaves, chopped
- Parmesan cheese
- Lemon juice
- Mint to sprinkle

Instructions

1. Heat the oven to 400 degrees Fahrenheit.
2. Add the fish to a tray with the lemon, salt and pepper and bake until soft.
3. Add the oil to a pan and allow it to heat.

4. Toss in the zucchini and squash along with the salt and pepper and mix until well combined.

5. Add in the fish by tearing it using a fork.

6. Add the balsamic and lemon juice on top and mix until well combined.

7. Add the Parmesan cheese and serve with a sprinkling of fresh mint leaves on top.

Lamb Patties with Mint Chutney

Ingredients

- 1 pound lamb, ground

- 1 tablespoon fresh rosemary, chopped

- 1 tablespoon coconut oil

- 1 bunch fresh basil leaves

- ¼ cup olive oil

- 1 teaspoon fresh lemon juice

- 1 clove of garlic, chopped

- ¼ cup sunflower seeds

- 2 cups mint

- 1 tablespoon olive oil

- 2 tablespoons white wine vinegar

- Salt to taste

- Pepper to taste

Instructions

1. Add the lamb, rosemary and salt to a bowl and mix until well combined.

2. Flatten it into patties.

3. Add the oil to a pan and place the patties on top.

4. Flip them over to brown on all sides.

5. Add the mint, seeds, olive oil, lemon and garlic to a processor and whizz.

6. Place the patties on a plate and top it with the mint chutney.

7. Serve hot.

Thai Salad

Ingredients

- Lettuce leaves, chopped
- Grilled Chicken, chopped
- Broccoli, chopped
- Mango and Cabbage Slaw
- Roasted Red Peppers, chopped
- Tomatoes, chopped

Chili vinaigrette

- 2 tablespoon rice vinegar
- 1 tablespoon olive oil
- 1 teaspoon fresh lime juice
- 1 teaspoon chili paste
- 1/2 teaspoon ginger, grated

Instructions

1. Prepare the vinaigrette by adding the vinegar, oil, lime, chili and ginger to a bowl and whisking until well combined.

2. Add the lettuce leaves, chopped chicken, broccoli, mango and cabbage slaw, tomatoes to a bowl and mix until well combined.

3. Drizzle the dressing on top and serve.

Chapter 13: Simple Paleo Dinner Recipes

Simple Chicken-Coconut Salad

Ingredients

- 1 small cabbage, chopped into slices

- 2 large carrots, chopped

- 1 tablespoon coconut oil

- 1/3 cup coconut flakes

- 1 tablespoon olive oil

- 2 garlic cloves, chopped

- 4 green onions, chopped

- ½ cup grilled chicken, shred

- Mint to sprinkle

Instructions

1. Add the oil to a pan and toss in the cabbage.

2. Mix until well combined.

3. Add in the carrots, and sauté until brown.

4. Toss in the garlic, onions and chicken and mix until well combined.

5. Add everything to a bowl along with the coconut flakes and chicken and mix until well combined.

6. Serve with a sprinkling of fresh mint leaves on top.

Broccoli Cashew Salad

Ingredients

- 3/4 Cup Roasted, Salted Cashews
- 5 1/2 tablespoon water
- 1 tablespoon Vinegar
- 4 teaspoon curry powder
- 2 1/2 teaspoon honey
- Salt to taste
- Pepper to taste

Salad

- 4 cups Broccoli, chopped
- 1/4 cup red onion, chopped
- 1/2 cup Cilantro, chopped
- 2 pieces grilled turkey, chopped
- 1/4 cup dried cranberries, chopped
- 2 tablespoon sunflower seeds
- 2 Tablespoon cashews, chopped
- Mint to sprinkle

Instructions

1. Add the cashews to a bowl along with the water and place in the fridge.

2. The next day, add it to a blender along with the water, vinegar, curry powder, salt, pepper and honey and whizz into a smooth paste.

3. Add the broccoli, onion, cilantro, cranberries, sunflower seeds and cashews and mix until well combined.

4. Drizzle the dressing on top and serve the salad with a sprinkling of fresh mint leaves on top.

Shrimp Salad

Ingredients

- 1 teaspoon garlic, chopped

- ½ pound raw shrimp, deveined

- ½ tablespoon butter

- ½ teaspoon chili powder

- ¼ teaspoon cayenne powder

- 1½ cups avocados, chopped

- 1 cucumber, sliced

- 4 cups spinach, chopped

Dressing

- 1-inch ginger, peeled

- 3 tablespoons oil

- 3 tablespoons lemon juice

- 2 tablespoons honey

- Salt to taste

- Pepper to taste

- Cilantro to sprinkle

Instructions

1. Add the butter to a skillet and allow it to heat.

2. Toss in the garlic and shrimp and sauté till crisp.

3. Add in chili and cayenne and mix until well combined.

4. The prawns should completely be coated in the chili.

5. Cut the avocado into bite sized pieces and add to a bowl.

6. Add in the chopped spinach leaves and mix.

7. Toss in the cooked shrimp and well combine.

8. To make the dressing, add the ginger, oil, lemon juice, honey, salt and pepper to a bowl and mix.

9. Drizzle the dressing on top and serve the salad with a sprinkling of fresh cilantro leaves on top.

Paleo Dinner Burgers

Ingredients

- 1½ beef, ground
- 1 teaspoon salt
- 1 teaspoon pepper
- 1 teaspoon garlic
- 2 tablespoons coconut oil
- 2 small onions, chopped
- 2 tablespoons balsamic vinegar
- 1 tomato, cut into circles
- 1 cup lettuce leaf, chopped into circles
- 3 avocados, chopped into circles

Instructions

1. Heat a pan and add in the coconut oil.
2. Once it heats toss in the beef, garlic and pepper.
3. Add in the vinegar and mix until well combined.
4. Make patties out of it and place on the same pan to brown on both sides.
5. To assemble the burger, place the tomato on a plate followed by the patties.

6. Place the lettuce leaves on top followed by the avocado slices.

Paleo Pizza

Ingredients

Crust

- 1 cup tapioca starch
- 1/4 cup coconut flour
- 2 eggs
- 1 cup water
- Salt to taste
- 2 tablespoons tomato paste

Toppings

- Prosciutto
- Fresh Tomatoes
- Jalapeños
- Spinach
- Onions
- Bell Peppers
- Fresh Basil

Instructions

1. Heat the oil in a pan and toss in the onions.

2. Once it browns, add in the chicken pieces, garlic, sunflower seeds and mix.

3. Add the salt, pepper and basil leaves and wait for everything to well combine.

4. Add in the coconut milk, tomatoes and water and mix until well combined.

5. Add the arrowroot powder to thicken the sauce.

6. Serve the curry hot with a sprinkling of fresh mint leaves on top. 7

Paleo Pork Chops

Ingredients

- 4 pork chops
- 1 teaspoon sea salt
- 1 teaspoon ground black pepper
- 2 tablespoons butter

Sauce

- 2 tablespoons balsamic vinegar
- 2 tablespoons honey
- 2 garlic cloves, chopped
- ½ teaspoon dried rosemary leaves
- ½ teaspoon dried oregano leaves
- 1 tablespoon red pepper flakes

Instructions

1. Preheat the oven to 400 degrees Fahrenheit.

2. Add the pork chops to a bowl along with the salt and pepper and mix until well combined.

3. Add the butter to a griddle and allow it to heat up.

4. Once it sizzles, add the pork to it and allow it to sizzle.

5. Meanwhile, add the vinegar, honey, and garlic to a pan and allow mixing well.

6. Add in the rosemary, oregano and pepper and mix until well combined.

7. Place the pork in the oven for 5 to 6 minutes or until crispy.

8. Add the dressing to it and return to heat.

9. Allow the sauces to stick to the pork and serve hot.

Chapter 14:
Simple Paleo Snack Recipes

Zucchini Chips

Ingredients

- 2 large zucchinis

- Salt to taste

- Pepper to taste

- Oil to apply

Instructions

1. Preheat the oven to 400 degrees Fahrenheit.

2. Cut the zucchini into thin circles.

3. Remember, the thinner they are, the faster they will crisp up.

4. Place them on a baking sheet and apply the oil on each piece.

5. Sprinkle the salt and pepper on top and place in the oven.

6. Allow them to crisp up on one side before flipping it over to the other.

7. Serve the chips warm.

Spicy Pumpkin Seeds

Ingredients

- 2 cups pumpkin seeds, dried

- 3 jalapeño peppers, chopped

- 3 tablespoons olive oil

- Sea salt to taste

- Paprika, to taste

Instructions

1. Dry the pumpkin seeds by placing them in the sun for a couple of days. If you have no time then microwave them for about 2 minutes.

2. Add them to a bowl along with the chopped jalapenos and mix until well combined.

3. Spread them over a baking tray and place in a preheated 350 degree Fahrenheit oven for 15 to 20 minutes or until crispy.

4. Serve hot with a sprinkling of salt and paprika on top.

Eggplant Chips

Ingredients

- 1 large eggplant

- 1/2 cup olive oil

- 5 tablespoons balsamic vinegar

- 2 tablespoons honey

- 1/2 teaspoon paprika powder

- Salt to sprinkle

Instructions

1. Preheat the oven to 350 degrees Fahrenheit.

2. Wash and slice the eggplants into thin long strips.

3. Add the vinegar, oil, and paprika, salt to a bowl and mix well.

4. Add the eggplants to the mix and marinate for5 to 6 hours.

5. Once they combine, place them on a greased baking tray and bake for 20 to 30 minutes or until crispy.

6. Serve warm.

Apple Nachos

Ingredients

- 2 green apples

- 2 tablespoon fresh lemon juice

- 1 tablespoon almond butter

- 2 tablespoons coconut shreds

- 2 tablespoons sliced almonds

Instructions

1. Slice the apples into thin slices and add to a bowl.

2. Add the lemon juice in and mix well.

3. Place the slices on a plate and drizzle the butter on top.

4. Serve with a sprinkling of freshly grated coconut on top.

Paleo Crackers

Ingredients

- 1 cup almond flour

- 1 large egg

- 1 tablespoon butter

- 1 teaspoon salt

Instructions

1. Preheat the oven to 350 degrees Fahrenheit.

2. Add the flour, egg, butter and salt to a bowl and whizz until well combined.

3. Once done, mold the batter into small circles and place on a baking tray.

4. Bake for 20 minutes or until the tops brown and the cookies bake through.

5. Serve warm.

Sweet Potato Chips

Ingredients

- 2 large sweet potatoes, peeled and chopped

- 1 tablespoon coconut oil, melted

- 1 teaspoon sea salt

- 2 teaspoon dried rosemary leaves

Instructions

1. Peel and chop the sweet potatoes into thin, long strips.

2. Preheat the oven to 400 degrees Fahrenheit.

3. Line the potato strips on a baking tray and apply the oil on top.

4. Sprinkle the salt and rosemary and place in the oven to crisp up.

5. Serve warm.

Filled Avocado

Ingredients

- 1/2 Avocado

- 1/3 Cup Greek Yogurt, beaten

- 1/2 teaspoon Paprika

- 1/2 teaspoon Salt

- 1/2 teaspoon Garlic Powder

Instructions

1. Scoop out the seed of an avocado and set aside.

2. Add the yogurt, paprika, salt and garlic to a bowl and mix until well combined.

3. Spoon the mixture in the center of the avocado.

4. Serve with a sprinkling of paprika on top.

Chapter 15:
Paleo Desserts

Lemon Pie Bars

Ingredients

- 1 cup almond flour
- 1/4 cup almond butter
- 1 tablespoon honey
- 1 tablespoon butter
- 1 teaspoon vanilla extract
- 1/2 teaspoon baking powder
- 1/4 salt to taste
- 3 eggs
- 1/2 cup honey
- 1/4 cup lemon juice
- 2 1/2 tablespoon coconut flour
- 1 tablespoon lemon zest, grated
- Salt to taste

Instructions

1. Preheat the oven to 350 degrees Fahrenheit.

2. Add the oil to a baking tray and spread.

3. Add the almond, butter, honey vanilla, salt and baking powder to a bowl and mix until well combined.

4. Press it onto the baking tray and place in the oven to brown.

5. Meanwhile, whisk together the eggs, honey, lemon juice, coconut flour, lemon zest and salt and mix until well combined.

6. Pour this mixture on top of the crust and place it back in the oven.

7. Allow it to cook for 10 minutes.

8. Serve by cutting into small squares.

Paleo Coconut Bars

Ingredients

- 4 cups grated coconut

- ½ cup melted coconut oil

- 4 tablespoons honey

- ¼ cup slivered almond

- 1½ cups dark chocolate pieces

Instructions

1. Add the coconut, coconut oil to a blender and whizz until smooth.

2. Add the honey to the mix and well combine.

3. Line a baking tray with grease and set aside.

4. Preheat the oven to 350 degrees Fahrenheit.

5. Add the coconut mix to the tray and spread it out evenly.

6. Sprinkle the almond on top and bake for 20 minutes or until the coconut browns.

7. Serve by cutting the mix into bite sized squares.

Paleo Doughnuts

Ingredients

- 2 cups almond meal
- 3/4 teaspoon baking soda
- 1/2 teaspoon salt
- 3 tablespoons coconut oil, melted
- 3 tablespoons honey, melted
- 1/2 teaspoon vanilla extract
- 3 teaspoons apple cider vinegar
- 3 large eggs

Instructions

1. Preheat the oven to 375 degrees Fahrenheit.
2. Add the coconut oil to a pan and melt.
3. Add the honey, vanilla, vinegar, melted oil and eggs to a bowl and whisk.
4. Add in the almond flour, salt and baking soda and mix until well combined.
5. Divide the batter into doughnut molds and bake for 12 to 15 minutes.
6. Serve warm.

Paleo Key Lime Pie

Ingredients

- 1 cup pecan nuts, soaked for a couple hours

- 1 cup almonds, soaked overnight

- 10 dates

- ¼ cup coconut oil

- ¼ teaspoon sea salt

For filling

- 5 medium avocados

- ¼ cup lime juice

- 1 tablespoon lime zest

- ½ cup coconut oil

- ½ cup raw honey

- 1 teaspoon vanilla extract

- ¼ teaspoon sea salt

Instructions

1. Add the crust ingredients to a bowl and mix until well combined.

2. Press the crust into molds and place in the freezer for 30 minutes to an hour.

3. Add the flesh of the avocados to the blender and whiz until smooth.

4. Mix in the lemon juice, lemon zest, coconut, honey, vanilla and salt and mix until well combined.

5. Spread this mixture on top of the crust and turn into the freezer for an hour.

6. Cut into slices and serve cold.

Paleo Cake

Ingredients

- ½ cup coconut flour
- 1½ cup tapioca starch
- 2 tablespoon cinnamon powder
- 3 teaspoon ginger powder
- 2 teaspoon allspice powder
- 1 teaspoon salt
- 2 pinches of cloves powder
- 2 teaspoon baking powder
- 1 cup butter
- 8 eggs
- 1 cup applesauce
- 1 cup coconut sugar
- 2 teaspoons vanilla extract
- 4 cups shredded carrot

Instructions

1. Preheat the oven to 350 degrees Fahrenheit.

2. Add the butter, eggs, applesauce, and vanilla extract to a bowl and whizz until well combined.

3. Run the coconut flour, starch, cinnamon and ginger powder, all spice, clove powder and baking powder through a sieve to well combine.

4. Mix the dry ingredients with the wet and mix well.

5. Add the mix to a baking tray and place in the oven to bake for 20 to 25 minutes.

6. Allow cooling before cutting and serving.

Paleo Cranberry Cookies

Ingredients

- 1 egg

- ½ cup almond butter

- ⅓ cup coconut sugar

- ½ teaspoon vanilla extract

- ¼ teaspoon baking soda

- ⅛ teaspoon salt

- ¼ cup cranberries, chopped

- ¼ cup chocolate chips

Instructions

1. Preheat the oven to 350 degrees Fahrenheit.

2. Add the egg to a bowl and beat.

3. Add in the rest of the ingredients and mix until well combined.

4. Make small cookies out of it and place on a greased baking tray.

5. Bake for 10 to 15 minutes or until brown on all sides.

Baked Banana

Ingredients

- 1 large banana
- 1 tablespoon butter
- ½ teaspoon cinnamon

Instructions

1. Preheat the oven to 375 degrees Fahrenheit.

2. Cut the bananas into halves.

3. Mix the butter and cinnamon in a bowl and add between the bananas.

4. Apply on the inner sides of the banana.

5. Bake for 10 minutes and serve warm.

Chapter 16:
Best Paleo Approved Foods

Spinach

Spinach is one of the topmost foods to include in your Paleo diet. It is rich in antioxidants and enhances good health. It is also known for its cancer-fighting benefits and immunity enhancing capacity. Spinach also assists in controlling sugar levels in the body thereby increasing resistance to diabetes. Spinach is rich in vitamins A, C, magnesium, and potassium. All of these contribute towards maintaining good health and increasing blood circulation in the body. Add spinach to salads and also makes for a great addition to curries and soups.

Kale

It is well known that kale helps in keeping both the body and mind fit. It is loaded with nutritional benefits all of which contribute towards maintaining a healthy body. In fact, it is believed that kale outdoes spinach regarding nutritional value provided. A cup of kale provides your body with higher doses of vitamin A and C. It also assists with adding back lost water and increases joint lubrication. It is, therefore, recommended to those suffering from arthritis and painful joints.

Avocado

Avocado is a great ingredient to add to your Paleo diet. The fruit is packed with nutrition and recommended to keep a tab on insulin secretion. The fruit is full of saturated fats that help in controlling bad cholesterol. It is also full of fiber that is meant to keep the digestive system in check. Cut up an avocado and dig away. It need not always be incorporated into a dish. But it is versatile enough to be added to a wide range of dishes including salads, soups, curries and also desserts.

Apples

It is no secret that apples are extremely healthy. They are full of antioxidants and other elements that are great for the body. The fiber content in apples is also regarded as one of the highest amongst fruits. Eat an apple every morning to maintain a slim body and keep illnesses at bay. Apples are known to prevent the onset of many types of cancers. It also assists with preventing the onset of Alzheimer's and so, makes for a great fruit to add to your regular diet.

Almonds

Almonds are one of the best snacking options. Not only do they fill you up, they also add multiple nutrients to your body. Just a handful can help to improve your overall health. Ground almond meal makes for a great substitute for a regular meal. Almond flour is also a great replacement for regular flour. It is used in cooking desserts such as cakes and also used as a thickening agent for soups and curries. Almonds are rich in vitamin E oils that enhance skin elasticity and enhance a youthful appearance.

Watermelon

Watermelon is one of the best natural ingredients to consume as per the Paleo diet as it is loaded with lycopene. Lycopene is known for its cancer-fighting benefits and enhances good health. Watermelon is a summer fruit but can be consumed the whole year round. It is rich in vitamin C and A, both of which assist in maintaining good health. Just cut up a few slices of watermelon and consume as a salad. It can also be juiced and consumed.

Fish

Freshwater fish such as salmon and trout are amazing fish to consume on a regular basis. It is filled with omega 3 fatty acids, which is responsible for keeping the heart and brain healthy. It is also easily digested and does not impose on the body. It can be incorporated in many different ways including adding to salads and curries. Fish oil makes for a great condiment and enhances flavor and health. It can be added to savory dishes to enhance the flavor and also uplift the taste of the dish.

Asparagus

Asparagus is just as loaded with multiple nutrients all meant to enhance good health and increase immunity. Just steam a few and consume it on a regular basis. They provide a crunch, which enhances the value of a dish. Asparagus helps in keeping the digestive system and also the urinary tract clean. It is also rich in fiber content thereby making it an ideal option for those looking to increase the fiber content in their meals.

Beetroots

Beetroots are not just colorful but also extremely healthy; they are full of antioxidants that strengthen the body from the inside. In fact, beetroots are extremely precious since they contain a unique and rare component known as Betalain, which is exclusively found in beets alone. This element detoxifies the body and cleanses the liver.

Chicken

Chicken is an important protein-rich ingredient in the diet. It is, in fact, one of the most preferred meats owing to its light quality and high protein content. It is better than red meats as they can be a little fatty. There are many ways to cook with chicken and does not have to be limited to grilling and roasting. It can be cooked and added to salads, curries, soups, etc. Chicken is also loaded with fiber thereby making it an ideal addition to everyday meals.

Lean beef

If you are too used to consuming red meats, then the best choice is lean beef. It is full of good proteins that enhance good health. It is also less in fatty content and will make for great diet ingredient. It is also great for hair and skin health as it contains a lot of vitamin B-12. Lean beef can be ground and made into patties. It is also a good ingredient to add to curries.

Eggs

No Paleo meal is complete without an egg. This is mainly because of the many health benefits that it provides. Right from giving your body a healthy dose of vitamin D and proteins, it also strengthens the core systems. Eggs are also very versatile and can be used in many different ways. Poaching one and adding to soups and curries is a great way to incorporate it into your meals.

Chapter 17:
Precautions/ Expectations

Before taking up the Paleo diet, there are a few basic precautions to bear in mind that are discussed as under.

Check up

Get a basic check up done before starting the diet. The doctor will check the different vital statistics before deciding on whether you make for a good candidate or not. Most individuals will get a clean chit, but there will be some that might have to wait until they turn likely candidates for the diet. Once you take up the diet, you can pay him a visit every few months to have it checked again and also check progress with the diet.

Supplements

The Paleo diet is great no doubt but can leave out some basic nutrients. The body cannot do without these and will be important to provide it with the same. These nutrients will help the body remain healthy and contribute towards optimal functioning. Some of them include vitamin D and calcium. This is not easily availed through the Paleo diet as it leaves out dairy products. A good way to make up for it will be by consuming supplements. Supplements will add these nutrients back to the body and enhance its functioning. Supplements need not always be chemical ones. There are natural supplements as well that can help the body in more or less the same way. Talk to your physician about it and ask him to suggest something natural.

Medications

If you are on any medications, then inform your doctor about the same and also tell him about the diet. Certain diets can tamper with the functioning of medication and will be important to have them checked. Your doctor will be able to prescribe alternatives that go well with the diet. If you consume supplements, then you must inform the doctor about the same.

Older people

It will be best for older people to exercise a little precaution when taking up the Paleo diet. The diet is mostly designed for people looking to lose weight, therefore, will leave out carbohydrates. Carbs will be required to maintain basic bodily functions and remain healthy. It leaves out a few important nutrients that are required by the body. Older people might need a little more of it to remain healthy. Some of the lost nutrients can be added back by consuming supplements, but older people might need additional dietary supplementation. It would, therefore, be best to consult a doctor first to ensure that the diet will be compatible.

Pregnant women

Pregnant and lactating women should also take precaution on a diet. Consult your doctor to know if it will be safe to take it up during pregnancy. The diet can leave out a few essential nutrients that might be important for your baby. If you were on a diet before getting pregnant, then it would be best to consult a doctor to know if it is feasible to continue with it. She might prescribe some supplements that can help with your health.

Children

Children can take up the Paleo diet. However, they might need supplements to keep them healthy. Calcium supplements will be a must to keep their bones strong. The diet is ideal for obese children. It will help them see quick results. But it should be supplemented with proper exercise. Get them to play more sports and time their meals well. If they do not see any substantial results with the diet, then discontinue it and reevaluate the diet.

Reasonable expectations

Once you take up the diet, you must have reasonable expectations from it. Some people end up having unreasonable ones and get disappointed. Don't set yourself high expectations and focus on something that is gettable. Your expectations should reflect on your body. If there are no positive signs, then it means you are pressurizing yourself too much. Step it down a little and give your body some time to adjust to the changes. If you are still unable to see results, then give it a break and restart once your body is ready.

Patience

You have to be patient when you take up a diet. Some people wish to see overnight results that are not feasible. Give yourself and your body some time to adapt to the changes and let the diet work its magic on you at its pace. If you try to hurry things up, then you will be disappointed. If things are not going to plan, then take it a little slow and reevaluate the steps that you have been taking. A few changes can go a long way in sustaining the diet and sticking with it in the long run.

Carbohydrates

Take it a little slow with reducing carbohydrate consumption, although the Paleo diet does not specify its reduction. The foods that it prescribes do not lend the body too many carbs. This can confuse your body initially. If you stop consuming it all together all at once, then you will find it difficult to keep up with the diet. You, therefore, must slow it down and go slow. Cravings are expected and will take some effort on your part to stave them off. It will come easy after the first few weeks, as that is when it will be hardest for you to control your cravings.

Comparisons

Do not compare your progress with that of others or even your partner. Everybody will see different results, and they will not be the same. Some might see faster results while some others might see slower ones. If you are not satisfied with your results, then look back at what you have been doing and how to fix the problem. But that should not discourage you from having a partner through the journey and pick someone that will keep at it with you.

Expenses

You might be surprised in the expense department. It will cost a lot lesser to take up the Paleo diet as you will eliminate consumption of junk and processed foods. However, it might be offset, to some extent, through the consumption of quality meats and organic foods. But it will be well worth the spending, as they will contribute towards maintaining your health. It will pay to set aside a budget for your diet. It will help with keeping a tab over your expenses and tell you exactly what you have spent the money on.

Cheat meals

Many diets allow consumption of cheat meals, as they can help with sticking better with the diet. However, the Paleo diet is extremely strict and will not allow the consumption of any cheat meals. You will not have the option of indulging in a burger or hot dog unless they are healthier versions that you have prepared yourself. A good idea is to prepare some of these treats at home, from time to time, and make it as tasty as possible. They will make for good replacements and satisfy your cravings.

Weakness

Weakness is a side effect of the diet that you must prepare for. This is only natural, especially if your body is used to a carbohydrate-rich diet. You might have to put up with a little weakness, especially after waking up. But that should not be a reason for you to stop with the diet. Keep a snack handy to munch on. It can be nuts or chopped up vegetables. They will put an end to the weakness.

Key takeaways

The Paleo diet came into limelight during the early 2000s and has since been viewed as one of the most preferred diets in the world. The diet is attributed to the work of many dieticians and doctors, all of who contributed towards shaping it into what it is today. The diet has gone through several modifications.

Modern day Paleo diet is more or less on par with what Paleo man followed, but for a few modifications. These modifications have been introduced bearing in mind the resources that are available in today's world and to make it easy for modern day dieters to take it up.

The Paleo diet relies on three basic food categories namely proteins, fruits, and vegetables, fats, and oils. All of these were freely available to Paleo man and thus, form a big part of the current diet.

The Paleo diet has been carved out to suit the palate of a wide range of people including vegetarians and non-vegetarians. Lean proteins, fresh fruits, and vegetables are the main components of the diet and make it one of the best ones to follow. However, it leaves out a long list of foods including junk, processed foods, whole grains, seeds, nuts, etc. All of these were not available to Paleo man and thus are not part of the diet. It is understood that most of us are used to consuming these on a regular basis but will have to be dropped for the Paleo diet.

The Paleo diet offers many health benefits. Right from keeping the heart healthy to maintaining skin and hair health, the diet offers a plethora of health benefits. Once you take it up, the results will fall into place, and you will begin to reel in a healthy body.

There are many reasons to take up the Paleo diet. Not only will it make you fitter and stronger but also allow you to lead a longer life filled with productivity. These form just some of the many other reasons that make the diet a great one to adopt. It is also one of the easiest to adopt thereby making it ideal for a wide range of people.

The diet is designed to mimic the food choices of Paleolithic man as he led a long healthy life. Although there is some misconception regarding the lifespan of Paleo man, he did lead a healthy life free from illnesses. The same can be channelized and adopted to lead a long life free from diseases brought about by modern day lifestyle choices.

The Paleo diet is easy to adopt and not as tough compared to some of the other diets in the world. You will be required to make just a few changes to your existing diet and be able to adopt it successfully. But it will be entirely up to you to keep up with the diet, as it is sometimes easy to fall out of a diet.

There are many things to do to stick with the diet. Overhauling your kitchen to incorporate Paleo friendly foods, investing in recipe books, picking a role model for yourself and joining a group can all help towards remaining put with the Paleo diet.

One of the biggest problems faced by those who take up the diet is not being able to go out with friends to a restaurant. Carrying your meals with you, however, can solve this issue. If that is not always possible, then look for a Paleo friendly salad on the menu and dig away!

There are many things to do during the diet to avail maximum benefit of it. Some of this includes staving off the temptation to overeat, skipping meals, not accounting liquid calories, cutting out fat immediately, etc. Making these changes will help you see faster results.

One of the main reasons for taking up the diet is to lose weight, but the only way in which that will work is if you team it up with some exercise. There are many routines to choose from including dancing, cardio exercises, and yoga. These will supplement the diet and give you better results.

The book provides you with a 1-week meal plan that will kick start your Paleo diet. All the dishes mentioned are easy to adopt and get you started on the right foot. These dishes can be switched up to your liking. For example, switch up the lunch options with the dinner options for the second week, the snack options with dinner options for the third, etc. They are quite flexible and can be adapted to your liking. Do not limit yourself to just these recipes and experiment with the ingredients to come up with some of your own.

We looked at the different super foods to consume as per the diet. They are filled with nutritional benefits and sure to enhance good health. Try to incorporate them into your diet as much as possible to develop a slim and lean body free from illnesses.

As is with any other diet, there are a few precautions to observe. These are basic ones meant to prepare you for the diet. Once you get the clean chit, it will be best to start with the diet immediately.

It is obvious that you will have a lot of expectations from the diet. Everybody takes it up to achieve one goal or another.

However, it will be best to have reasonable expectations out of the diet. Unreasonable expectations will only lead to disappointment and so, will be best to sketch out a reasonable expectation plan before starting out with the diet.

It is vital for you to be patient when you take up the Paleo diet. Take it slow if it is a bit daunting. Once you settle in, it will get progressively easier.

Conclusion

I thank you once again for choosing this book and hope you had a fun time reading it.

The main aim of this book was to educate you on the basics of the Paleo diet and what taking it up can do for your health. I have done my bit by giving you the steps and strategies to adopt. It is now up to you to put them to practice.

Once you take up the diet, the positive effects that it has on your body will surprise you. After seeing these results you will want to continue the diet for a lifetime. All it takes is a little perseverance, and you will have the chance to attain the body of your dreams.

If you liked this book, then please share it with others in your life who can benefit from the Paleo diet. You can also introduce it to your children, as they can start early and mold their bodies. You don't have to stick to the recipes mentioned in this book and develop some of your own. Mix and match the ingredients to make dishes that fit in well with your palate.

I wish you luck with your diet and hope you see positive results.

Good luck!

References

https://www.hsph.harvard.edu/nutritionsource/omega-3-fats/

http://umm.edu/health/medical/altmed/supplement/omega3-fatty-acids#ixzz3BpvtzHsG

http://www.health.harvard.edu/fhg/updates/What-you-eat-can-fuel-or-cool-inflammation-a-key-driver-of-heart-disease-diabetes-and-other-chronic-conditions.shtml

https://www.choosemyplate.gov/vegetables

http://www.nutritionletter.tufts.edu/issues/10_2/current-articles/Discover-the-Digestive-Benefits-of-Fermented-Foods_1383-1.html

https://www.hsph.harvard.edu/obesity-prevention-source/obesity-causes/diet-and-weight/

https://www.ncbi.nlm.nih.gov/pmc/articles/PMC2787021/

www.ingramcontent.com/pod-product-compliance
Lightning Source LLC
Chambersburg PA
CBHW070140290526
45789CB00002B/564